MW01226642

Keto Bread Cookbook

Table of content

Introduction

Bread is one of the basics of life, from the rolls and dumplings to the loaves of bread to specialty breads, there's no end to the ways you can enjoy bread in your day. You know that bread is the little touch you need with your soup, as a side to your dinner, or even as a little snack to get you through the afternoon.

But, you also know how hard you have been trying to stick with your diet. From all the carbs you count to the gluten you avoid, or the paleo foods you are so careful to monitor, it just doesn't seem like bread is going to fit on the menu.

So what do you do? Do you spend your life without bread and suffer through with only lettuce or other leaves as wraps? Do you look at the soup you have made and think about how bread would be next to it?

But, you go ahead and stick with your diet in spite of the fact you really want that bread, and you trudge through your day, but not nearly as happy as you could be. After all, you know you love the scale when you see that your diet is working, but when you are standing in the kitchen it's hard to stick with a diet that doesn't allow you to have staples like bread.

Thankfully, that's all over now. With this book, you have discovered what you need to still enjoy your bread though you are on a specialty diet. This book is full of breads and muffins and other wonderful loaves that will rock your day while you stay on track.

There's no end to the different ways you can use bread in your day, and with this cookbook, you will have your bread whenever you want, and however you want.

I'm going to show you just what you need to do to get the breads that match your needs, and help you enjoy bread like you once did. You will stick with your diet, you will still lose the weight that you wish to lose, and you will get to enjoy your bread as you once did.

Let me unlock the specialty bread recipes that will fit seamlessly into your specialty diet, and you can dive into the breads and other bread products you once enjoyed.

Open up the door to all the breads you could possibly ask for, and enjoy all your meals as you once did.

Just because you are on a specialty diet doesn't mean that you can't still enjoy breads as you once did, you just have to be creative about it. This book is going to show you all that and then some, so preheat your oven.

Let's get started.

Chapter 1 – So You Thought You Could Live a Life Without Bread?

Choosing a diet that's right for you can be excessively difficult, especially when you love so many foods that are suddenly placed on the "off limits" list.

But, there is a struggle there as you fight to find the diet that is right for you, that will give you the results that you are craving, and that will fit into the lifestyle you currently live. Because, though you know you should probably make some changes here and there, and if you are going to achieve the results you hope for, it's going to require you do give up on some of the things you love.

This all seems really easy, and even easier when you see the results starting to show. Suddenly, the numbers on the scale begins to drop, your clothes are fitting you differently, and you feel better than ever. Perhaps you are even sleeping better and getting sick less often.

Whatever your goals are, you can see that with the little changes you have made, you are getting closer to achieving those goals.

But then reality sets in.

Our diets... both as a society and branching out into the global world, revolves strongly around bread and bread products in one way or another.

Of course when you think about the foods you are giving up for a new diet, bread is rarely on the list right away.

There are a lot of foods you suddenly can't have, no matter how badly you want them. Though on the outset of the diet you didn't think you were going to miss certain foods, now that you can't have them anymore, it seems like the hardest thing in the world.

You see these foods everywhere, and suddenly the list of foods you now consider staples feel tasteless and bland. You simply must get your hands on some of that food from your past but you don't sacrifice the changes you have already made in order to do it.

You know bread is on this list. You loved bread, and though you thought it was going to be simple to give it up, it wasn't long before you realized that bread is a large enough staple in your day, you now can't imagine a life without it, and you would do anything to be able to enjoy it again.

From bread on the side of dinner to bread being the main course, suddenly, bread is all you can think about and the only thing that sounds good.

But bread is loaded with carbs and gluten, things you are supposed to be avoiding. This puts you at a cross roads. You know what you want, but you are also dedicated to your diet, and you don't want to stress about cheating on that.

But you are dying for that loaf of bread, and it doesn't seem as though there is any way you are going to get it.

Don't misunderstand me, I am aware that many people have tried their hand at making gluten free bread, and that there are many, many options on the market today.

Perhaps you have tried your hand at grain free bread making before. As you are aware, there are many people who feel the same way about this as you do, and they are going to do whatever they can to remedy the situation. But, when it comes to baking bread the untraditional way, you are bound to run into your fair share of issues.

Many different grain free breads are dry and crumbly, and they tend to have a flat flavor. Many also call for foods that aren't exactly considered to be real food, meaning you have to compromise in your diet plan in another way if you want the bread.

9

The secret to the success of your grain free bread lies in both the quality of the ingredients you use, as well as the type of ingredients you use.

In other words, don't be afraid to use real, and experiment with what works for you.

As you will see, the recipes in this book rely heavily on coconut flour. Coconut flour is an incredible option if you want something that is light and easy to work with, don't overpower the bread with a lot of its own flavor, and something you can find easily.

Yes, it's true that many people have complained that their coconut flour tends to make the bread dry, but this isn't an issue with the flour itself, but rather, how the flour is being used. When it comes to using the flour, you have to compensate with other ingredients, in this case, eggs.

Eggs are an excellent way to bring in moisture and buoyancy to your breads without weighing it down with carbs, sweeteners, or anything that goes against what you want to do for yourself.

As you work your way through the recipes in this book, you are going to notice that eggs and coconut flour are present in most, and that the amount of eggs you use is going to be directly affected by the amount of coconut flour in the recipe.

10

However, even when it comes to such things as coconut flour, coconut oil, and coconut milk, you do have freedom. Choose another kind of flour if you like, or try blending flours or using different kinds of oils.

Bear in mind the changes you make are going to affect the flavor of the bread, but for many, the different results add variety and gives them more options with their grain free lifestyle.

All in all, there is going to be a level of trial and error with any recipe you try, especially when you are working with food that has been traditionally prepared a certain way for centuries, but things are constantly growing and changing, and your bread is no exception.

Indulge in all these recipes, and have fun modifying them and turning them into your own. You know you have missed bread, and now is your chance to bring it back into your life not only occasionally, but as often as you want.

Let's get started.

Chapter 2 – Traditional Loaves

You reach a point when any bread is going to do, and you would do just about anything to get your hands on a loaf that will serve the purpose you need. But, you also know that you have high expectations, and bread that is falling apart or bread that is coarse and tasteless just isn't going to cut it.

These are traditional breads that you can use for anything you ever wanted bread for. Sandwiches, toast, dry them and make croutons… and the list goes on. Learn how to make the basic loaf of bread, and you will open the door to most things bread that you want to make in the future.

Now remember, I did say that trial and error is going to come into play here, and it's true. As much as you want your bread right now, you might have to make due with some loaves that aren't as good as you want them to be at first. But trust me, these recipes are delicious and yield excellent results, so stick with it until you get what you're after.

Sandwich Loaves

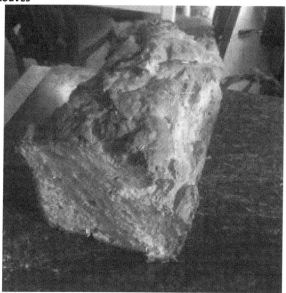

What you will need:

1 ½ cup milk

4 packets stevia

2 teaspoons dry active yeast

3 cups coconut flour

1 ½ teaspoon xanthan gum

4 teaspoons baking powder

1 teaspoon Himalayan sea salt

2 teaspoons apple cider vinegar

3 eggs

Directions:

In a bowl, combine the milk, stevia, and the yeast. Warm this in the microwave slightly, until you can put your finger into the mix and it's warm, but not hot.

Combine the rest of the ingredients in another mixing bowl, using a hand mixer.

Make sure that your yeast as sat for 10 minutes, then combine this to the rest of the mix, mixing well. The dough is going to be wet and sticky, but it's also going to be very thick.

Prepare your bread pan by lining it with parchment paper, or by spraying it with a bit of no stick cooking spray.

Scoop the mix into your bread pan and smooth out the top. Cover and set on top of your stove to rise as you preheat your oven.

Preheat the oven to 350 degrees F. Let your bread rise on top of the stove for 25 minutes, then place in the oven. Bake for 30-45 minutes, until the crust is a nice golden brown color.

Remove from pan immediately, and let cool on the counter.

Gluten Free Dinner Bread

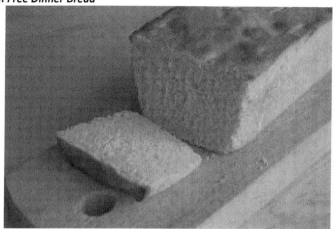

What you will need:

3 packets stevia

1 packet active dry yeast

1 ¼ cup warm water

2 cups coconut flour

½ cup cornstarch

½ cup potato starch

1/3 cup coconut oil

4 eggs

1 tablespoon xanthan gum

Dash of salt

Directions:

Combine the yeast and the stevia in a bowl of warm water.

In another mixing bowl, combine all the dry ingredients first, then add the wet ingredients.

Spray a loaf pan with no stick spray, then use a wooden spoon to spoon the dough into the loaf pan.

Let the dough rise in the pan until it has just reached above the edge of the pan. This is going to take roughly an hour.

Preheat your oven to 375 degrees F while the dough rises, then bake in the oven for 25 minutes, or until the loaf is golden brown.

Remove from the pan, then let cool on the counter.

Sweet Bundt Bread

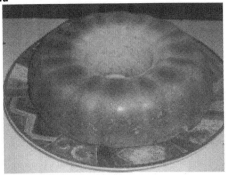

What you will need:

1 ½ cup milk

4 packets stevia, plus 6 packets stevia

2 teaspoons dry active yeast

3 cups coconut flour

1 ½ teaspoon xanthan gum

4 teaspoons baking powder

1 teaspoon Himalayan sea salt

2 teaspoons apple cider vinegar

4 eggs

Directions:

In a bowl, combine the milk, 4 packs of stevia, and the yeast. Warm this in the microwave slightly, until you can put your finger into the mix and it's warm, but not hot.

Combine the rest of the ingredients in another mixing bowl, using a hand mixer.

Make sure that your yeast as sat for 10 minutes, then combine this to the rest of the mix, mixing well. The dough is going to be wet and sticky, but it's also going to be very thick.

Prepare your bread pan by lining it with parchment paper, or by spraying it with a bit of no stick cooking spray.

Scoop the mix into your bread pan and smooth out the top. Cover and set on top of your stove to rise as you preheat your oven.

Preheat the oven to 350 degrees F. Let your bread rise on top of the stove for 25 minutes, then place in the oven. Bake for 30-45 minutes, until the crust is a nice golden brown color.

Remove from pan immediately, and let cool on the counter.

Chapter 3 – Do You Know the Muffin Man?

The traditional breads certainly have their place, but what about when you need a muffin, or you are just dying for a pancake or a waffle? With this chapter, you are going to get a taste of some of the old bread products you fell in love with, but have had to sacrifice for your specialty diet.

Feel free to change up the fruit you use in the muffins, there's no end to the ways you can satisfy that muffin craving.

Cranberry Muffins

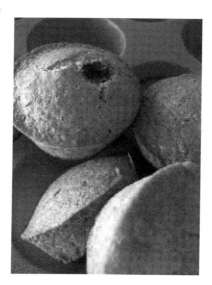

What you will need:

1 large egg

¼ cup coconut oil

1 large mashed banana

2 packets stevia

½ teaspoon salt

1 ½ teaspoons baking soda

1 teaspoon cinnamon

½ cup coconut milk

2/3 cup gluten free rolled oats

1 cup dried cranberries

1 ½ cup coconut flour

Directions:

Combine the dry ingredients in a mixing bowl, then add the wet ingredients next. Set aside.

Preheat your oven to 375 degrees F. and as your oven preheats, line your muffin tins with muffin liners. Spoon the batter into each of these cups, filling them most of the way but not entirely to the top.

Place in the oven and bake for 30-40 minutes. They will turn a deep golden brown color, and be firm to the touch. You will know when they are done when you can insert a toothpick into the center and it comes out clean.

Roll out onto a rack to cool, and enjoy!

World's Best Gluten Free Waffles

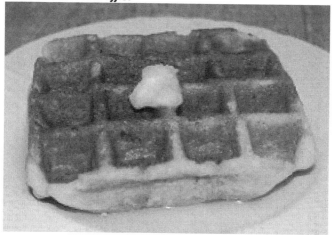

What you will need:

2 cups coconut flour

2 teaspoons baking powder

1 packet stevia

1 tablespoon coconut oil

Dash of salt

Splash of vanilla

4 eggs

Directions:

Spray your waffle iron with no stick cooking spray, and preheat. Combine all ingredients in a mixing bowl, then spoon generously onto your waffle iron.

Cook according to the waffle iron's directions, and serve hot.

All Purpose Gluten Free Naan

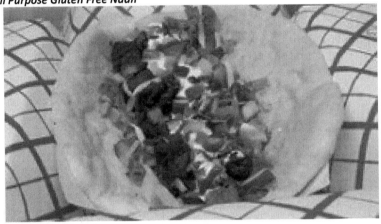

What you will need:

2 cups coconut flour

Splash of milk

2 teaspoons baking powder

1 packet stevia

1 tablespoon coconut oil

Dash of salt

Splash of vanilla

4 eggs

Directions:

Spray a griddle with no stick cooking spray, and heat over medium heat on the stove.

Scoop the batter onto the griddle, cooking for only a few minutes on each side. the bread is going to cook quickly, so keep an eye on it and flip it often.

Let cool before serving.

Chapter 4 – Taste of Italy

Pizza makes the world go round, and it certainly does its part in bringing the world together, but when it comes to a gluten free pizza crust, you are often left with a cracker that's so dry you don't want it.

These are rich and tasty crusts with a chewiness to them that is sure to satisfy your true pizza craving. Suddenly, pizza night is a normal thing once again, and your only limit is how many toppings you can fit on top.

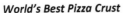
World's Best Pizza Crust

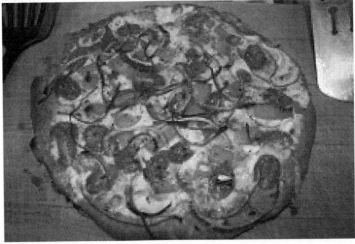

What you will need:

1 cup coconut flour

1 cup almond flour

1 cup tapioca flour

1 teaspoon xanthan gum

3 teaspoons salt

3 packets stevia

2 packets yeast

1 ½ cups warm water

1 tablespoon olive oil

½ teaspoon baking powder

Directions:

Combine all the dry ingredients first, then add in the wet ingredients after. Mix with a wooden spatula, combining all the ingredients well. You must be careful to ensure that all is mixed completely and don't let the water make the flour clump.

Once all ingredients are mixed, grease a pizza pan with no stick cooking spray, and lay the dough on next. You will have to use your fingers to ensure that it all spreads evenly across the pan, and that there are no thick or thin places.

Preheat your oven to 350 degrees, and pre-bake the crust for 10 minutes.

Let the crust sit for a few minutes before adding the toppings of your choice, then bake in the oven for an additional 20 minutes.

Enjoy!

Flat Bread Pizza Crust

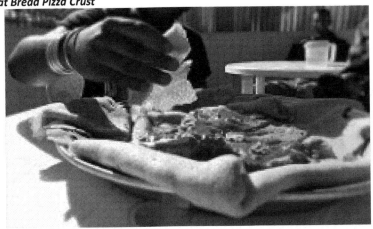

What you will need:

1 cup coconut flour

1 cup almond flour

1 cup tapioca flour

1 teaspoon xanthan gum

3 teaspoons salt

3 packets stevia

1 teaspoon Italian seasoning

1 tablespoon olive oil

½ teaspoon baking powder

Directions:

Combine all the dry ingredients first, then add in the wet ingredients after. Mix with a wooden spatula, combining all the ingredients well. You must be careful to ensure that all is mixed completely and don't let the water make the flour clump.

Once all ingredients are mixed, grease a pizza pan with no stick cooking spray, and lay the dough on next. You will have to use your fingers to ensure that it all spreads evenly across the pan, and that there are no thick or thin places.

Preheat your oven to 350 degrees, and pre-bake the crust for 10 minutes.

Let the crust sit for a few minutes before adding the toppings of your choice, then bake in the oven for an additional 20 minutes.

Enjoy!

Garlic Breadsticks

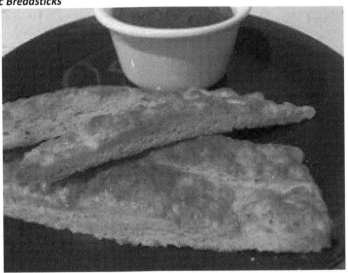

What you will need:

1 cup coconut flour

1 cup almond flour

1 cup tapioca flour

1 teaspoon xanthan gum

3 teaspoons salt

3 packets stevia

2 packets yeast

1 ½ cups warm water

1 tablespoon olive oil

½ teaspoon baking powder

1 tablespoon garlic powder

Cheese, if desired

Directions:

Combine all the dry ingredients first, then add in the wet ingredients after. Mix with a wooden spatula, combining all the ingredients well. You must be careful to ensure that all is mixed completely and don't let the water make the flour clump.

Once all ingredients are mixed, grease a pizza pan with no stick cooking spray, and lay the dough on next. You will have to use your fingers to ensure that it all spreads evenly across the pan, and that there are no thick or thin places.

Take a fork and stab holes into the dough at various intervals, to help the dough remain even through the baking.

Preheat your oven to 375 degrees, and pre-bake the crust for 25-30 minutes.

If you would like, sprinkle a bit of cheese on the top, and you are done!

Enjoy!

Chapter 5 – The Best of the Rest of the Breads

Dinner rolls, banana bread, corn bread. Oh those little sides that you don't miss until they are gone! Now, you can have each of them back in style with these gluten free and low carb options.

Your chili is going to have corn bread again, your meatloaf is going to have dinner rolls. There's simply no end to the dinners you can make to be what they used to be, helping you stay on track with your diet once again.

With these recipes, you can continue on your diet as you always have, and continue to see the benefits that you have worked so hard for, but you don't have to sacrifice on the meals you love to do it.

Enjoy these side dish breads, and embellish those meals you loved once again. Just sit back and ask someone to pass the rolls.

Gluten Free Dinner Rolls

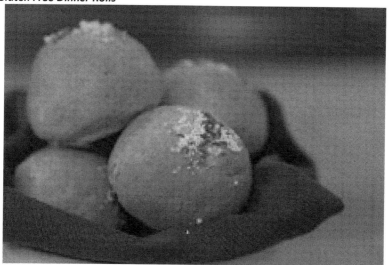

What you will need:

3 packets stevia

1 packet active dry yeast

1 ¼ cup warm water

2 cups coconut flour

½ cup cornstarch

½ cup potato starch

1/3 cup coconut oil

4 eggs

1 tablespoon xanthan gum

Dash of salt

Optional: You can add Italian seasoning or garlic to these rolls for a bit of added flavor depending on the dish you are making. If you choose to add either one, simply add a 2 teaspoons to a tablespoon to taste.

Directions:

In another mixing bowl, combine all the dry ingredients first, then add the wet ingredients.

Spray a 9 x 13 inch baking pan with no stick spray, then grease your hands with no stick spray.

Break off pieces of the dough from the main loaf and roll into balls in your hand, then lay them in the loaf pan. You should be able to get 24 rolls with this recipe, but you can adjust the size of the rolls for the amount you need.

Let the dough rise in the pan until it has just reached above the edge of the pan. This is going to take roughly an hour.

Preheat your oven to 375 degrees F while the dough rises, then bake in the oven for 25 minutes, or until the rolls is golden brown.

Remove from the pan, then let cool on the counter.

Once cooled, use your hands or a butter knife to gently pull the rolls apart, then stack in a basket on a clean bread cloth and serve!

Sultry Corn Bread

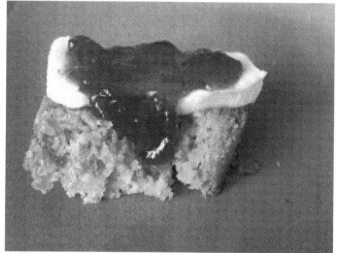

What you will need:

1 cup gluten free cornmeal

½ cup sweet rice flour

4 packets steviae

½ cup coconut flour

1 tablespoon baking powder

½ teaspoon salt

¼ teaspoon xanthan gum

3 large eggs

½ cup coconut milk

2 tablespoons butter (or a vegan butter alternative)

Directions:

You will need an 8 inch by 8 inch baking pan. Lightly grease with gluten free no stick cooking spray, and preheat your oven to 350 degrees F.

Start by mixing the dry ingredients in a large bowl, using a whisk to blend them together after the addition of each new ingredient. Then add the eggs in, one at a time. After the eggs have been mixed in, add the rest of the wet ingredients, and mix well.

Place the cornbread in the oven and bake for 30 to 35 minutes. The top of the cornbread will turn a golden brown, and you should be able to insert a toothpick into the center and have it come out clean.

Remove from the oven when the cornbread is finished cooking, and place on a wire rack to cool.

Cut into even squares when serving, and enjoy.

Nutty Banana Bread

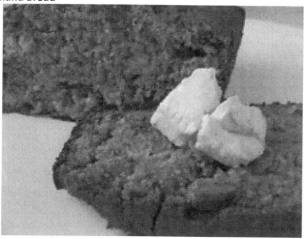

What you will need:

2 cups coconut flour

5 very ripe bananas

4 packets stevia

½ cup vegan butter alternative

2 eggs

2 tablespoons coconut milk

Splash of vanilla

1 teaspoon baking powder

1 teaspoon baking soda

Pinch of Himalayan Sea Salt

½ cup crushed walnuts

½ cup crushed pecans

Directions:

Start by preheating your oven to 350 degrees, and grease a loaf pan. I use a normal loaf pan for this, but feel free to experiment with different shapes and sizes.

Combine the dry ingredients in a large bowl, whisking them all together one at a time.

In another bowl, use your hand mixer to cream together the butter alternative with the milk, vanilla, and eggs.

Mash the bananas with a fork on a plate, mashing them until they are nearly a liquid. Add these to the wet ingredients and blend well.

Add all wet ingredients to the dry ingredients next, mixing well. Once you are certain there are no lumps in the batter, transfer into your loaf pan, smoothing the top.

Bake in the oven for 50 minutes to an hour, keeping an eye on it while it bakes. The top will be a nice golden brown, and a toothpick inserted into the center must come out clean.

Allow to cool for an hour before serving, then slice and enjoy!

Conclusion

There you have it, a complete collection of low carb, paleo friendly, gluten free breads that you can make and serve for a variety of meals or occasions. As you saw, each of the recipes in this book are incredibly easy to follow, and most of them are also incredibly inexpensive to make.

These breads are made using the normal ingredients you can find locally, so there's no need to have to order anything, or have to go to any specialty stores for any of them. With these breads, you can enjoy the same meals you used to enjoy, but stay on track with your diet as much as you want.

Lose the weight you want to lose, feel great, and still get to indulge in that piping hot piece of bread every now and then. Spread on your favorite topping, and your bread craving will be satisfied.

I hope the recipes in this book were able to inspire you to take your own baking to the next level. As you can see by each of these, you can alter and modify a variety of things to give them that custom spin you need from time to time. Sure, you might need to add garlic to this recipe or Italian seasoning to that.

You might want to substitute a nut for a fruit or different kinds of fruits within the recipe. Double the recipe, or cut it in half. There's no end to the ways you can indulge your bread desires, and with the recipes in this book, you will get the moist, consistent results you have been hoping for.

So many times gluten free bread ends up dry, and you don't want that. You want something that is as soft and pliable as the bread you are used to having. You want something that you can enjoy without fear that it's going to break apart the moment you pick it up, or that your guests are going to find it dry.

When it comes to your diet, you want only the best, and that's exactly what these breads are. From the accent rolls you can serve with your main dish to the waffles you can serve as your main dish, this book is full of the recipes you need to get through your day on your specialty diet.

Recommend the recipes to your friends who have no dietary restrictions, and show them just how tasty your way of eating really is. Dispel any myths about gluten free bread, and dive into a new way of cooking that's going to change your life.

Are you ready to enjoy those breads as you once did? Are you ready to serve soup or salad with a side of breadsticks or rolls? Are you ready to have a pizza night once again?

You know you are, so what are you waiting for? Grab your apron and preheat your oven. All you need is a few simple ingredients and your mixing bowl, and your set to have your bread and eat it, too.

FREE Bonus Reminder

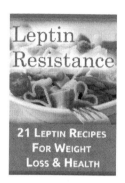

If you have not grabbed it yet, please go ahead and download your special bonus report *"Leptin Resistance. 21 Leptin Recipes For Weight Loss & Healthy Living"*.

Simply Click the Button Below

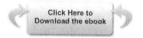

OR **Go to This Page**

http://easyweightlossway.com/free/

BONUS #2: More Free Books

Do you want to receive more Free Books?

We have a mailing list where we send out our new Books when they go free on Kindle. Click on the link below to sign up for Free Book Promotions. => Sign Up for Free Book Promotions <=

OR Go to this URL http://bit.ly/1V4Xan7

Made in the USA
Middletown, DE
26 September 2018